ENDOMETRIOSIS DIET & COOKBOOK

EVERYTHING YOU NEED TO KNOW ABOUT ENDOMETRIOSIS, TREATMENTS, AND DIET PLANS TO LEAD A PRODUCTIVE LIFE

BY

CAILIN CHASE

Contents

INTRODUCTION 1
CHAPTER ONE ARE YOU A VICTIM OF ENDOMETRIOSIS? 2
- *Painful periods:* 2
- *Excessive bleeding:* 2
- *Pain during sex:* 2
- *Rectal bleeding:* 3
- *Infertility:* 3
- *Other symptoms:* 3

CAUSES OF ENDOMETRIOSIS 4
THE AFFECTED AREAS: 4
OVARIAN CANCER: 4

CHAPTER TWO HOW TO PREVENT ENDOMETRIOSIS 5
NATURAL THERAPIES: 5
   Dietary changes 5
CASTOR OIL RECOMMENDATION 5
USE OF COMBINED CONTRACEPTIVES: 5
   Exercise: 5
   Usage of birth control pills: 6
   Intake of naproxen: 6
   Surgical removal: 6
   Hormonal therapy: 7

CHAPTER THREE HEALTH RECIPES TO PREVENT ENDOMETRIOSIS 8
CHOCOLATE CHEESECAKE 9
   Ingredients: 9
   Crust: 9
   Method: 9
HOT CHOCOLATE 10
   Ingredients: 10
   Method: 10
SCRUMPTIOUS HALIBUT PASTA 11
   Ingredients: 11
   Sauce: 11
   Method: 11

SNOWBALL TRUFFLES 12
   Ingredients: 12
METHOD: 12
   Ingredients: 13
   Method: 13
APRICOT AND CHOCOLATE MOUSSE 15
   Ingredients: 15

Method:	15
PIE PASTRY	16
Ingredients:	16
Method:	16
AMBROSIAL VEGETABLE PIE	17
Ingredients:	17
Method:	17
DOUBLE CHOCOLATE MUD PIES	18
Ingredients:	18
Double chocolate:	18
Method:	18
PRESTO PESTO	19
Ingredients:	19
TWO NUT FREE CARAMELS	20
Ingredients:	20
Chocolate:	20
Method:	20
CHOCOLATE CARAMELS	21
Method:	21
CHAPTER FOUR TIPS FOR HAPPINESS AND PRODUCTIVITY	**22**
Don't tolerate negative thoughts:	22
Live in the moment:	22
Enjoy every bit of your life:	23
Focus on the strengths you have:	23
Get to know yourself:	23
Take care of your needs:	23
Meditate:	23
Work with your fears:	24
Let go of the past:	24
Smile:	24
Do less:	24
Slow down:	24
Get organized:	24
Simplify your finances:	24
Do not compare yourself to others:	25
Learn to lose arguments:	25
Enjoy the little things:	25
CHAPTER FIVE WHY DO PEOPLE GAIN WEIGHT?	**26**
THE GENETICS THEORY:	26
THE ENVIRONMENT THEORY:	26
THE FAT CELL THEORY:	27
THE BROWN FAT THEORY:	27
THE ENZYME THEORY:	27
THE SET POINT THE THEORY:	28

CARBOHYDRATE BALANCE THEORIES: 28

CHAPTER SIX HOW TO LOSE WEIGHT? 30

    EAT HEALTHY: 32
    EXERCISE: 32
    DRINK WATER: 32
    SLEEP: 32
    WAIT UNTIL YOUR STOMACH RUMBLES BEFORE YOU REACH THE FOOD: 32
    EAT IN FRONT OF MIRRORS: 32
    WALK: 32
    ORDER THE SMALLEST PORTION OF EVERYTHING: 33
    EAT MINIMUM IN YOUR DINNER: 33

CHAPTER SEVEN SIMPLIFICATION IN LIFE 34

    LIMIT YOU'RE COMMUNICATIONS: 35
    ACCEPTANCE OF WHAT YOU HAVE: 35
    COMPLAIN LESS: 35
    LEARN TO SAY NO: 36
    DON'T MEDDLE IN OTHER PEOPLE'S BUSINESS. 36
    ENJOY WITHOUT OWNING. 36

CHAPTER EIGHT A GOAL IN LIFE 37

CHAPTER NINE ENJOY THE JOURNEY 39

    Release the need for immediate results: 40
    Fall in love with the journey: 40

CHAPTER TEN DEVELOP INTIMATE RELATIONSHIPS 41

- *Emotional intimacy:* 41
- *Spiritual intimacy:* 41
- *Physical intimacy:* 41
- *Work intimacy:* 41
- *Crisis intimacy:* 42
- *Intellectual intimacy:* 42

    HOW TO BUILD AND MAINTAIN A FAITHFUL RELATIONSHIP? 42
    PAY ATTENTION TO YOUR PARTNER IN THE EARLY STAGE: WHEN WE START BUILDING A 42
    Overt criticism in a relationship: 42
    Share mutual goals and plans with your partner: 43
    Equal give and take interaction: 43
    Balance in life: 43

CHAPTER ELEVEN EXERCISE-AN IMPORTANT THING IF LIFE 44

    Prevent diseases: 44
    Improves stamina: 44
    Strengthens and tones: 44
    Increases flexibility: 45
    Controls weight: 45

Improves quality of life:	*45*
Improved sex life:	*45*
You will live longer:	*45*
Lowers Type 2 diabetes risk.	*45*
Maintains immune functioning.	*45*
Reduces the risk of ARTHRITIS The	*46*
Boosts	*46*
Lowers	*46*
AEROBIC EXERCISE	47
CONCLUSION	**48**

Description

This reliable little book contains the most recent research on endometriosis, its causes, and symptoms and how to cure it. It includes all the stages of that disease and the other diseases that are affiliated to it. It also contains the recent research on effective weight loss and weight maintenance.

"What is Endometriosis and How to Live Productive Life without Pain through Diet and Exercise" dispels the myths and presents only the facts. Its sound, practical advice comes from health-care professionals you can trust.

And their information can help you improve your odds for a longer and healthier life.

Concise and clearly learning, "What is Endometriosis and How to Live Productive Life without Pain through Diet and Exercise" is a must reading for everyone interested in better health or get rid of Endometriosis.

Keep it handy. You'll refer to it often.

INTRODUCTION

Many people don't know what endometriosis is. It is a scientific disorder which lasts long and is found in women. There is an abnormal growth of the tissues (endometrial cells) on the outer side of the uterus instead of the inner surface. Endometrial cells are the cells that cover the uterus and sheds off every month during menstruation. Millions of women across the globe are the victim of this disease. It does not affect the menstrual cycle in any way because the grown misplaced tissues develop in the same way that the tissues of the uterine lining does: each month the tissue build up, breaks down and sheds. This is immensely painful and disturbing.

Life could be spent very productively without distress through regular exercise and a healthy diet. Eating poorly and not exercising could be taking a toll on areas other than your waistline -- it could also affect how productive you are at work, new research suggests. In "What is Endometriosis and How to Live Productive Life Without Pain Through Diet and Exercise", you will also learn about the scientific basis for obesity, the current treatment methods, and how to plan a weight control program with the help of exercise and diet only. The health risk associated with being overweight is also discussed. The most solid aspects of wellness that fit strongly in the realm of medicine are the environmental health, nutrition and the disease prevention that can be investigated and assist in measuring well-being. Hence both these elements are considered as important points to lead a happy life. This book does not come with a money back guarantee that you will lose weight, but, this book provides the tools necessary to make a weight loss program work for you and the essential elements to lead a contended life.

Chapter one Are you a victim of endometriosis?

Why did I get endometriosis? Why me? Many of us that are victims of this horrible and debilitating disease want to know why and how we got it in the first place. Unfortunately, Endometriosis is not a disease with a single cause. Many clinicians have long been attempting to find the key to the onset of endometriosis. Further probing brought up other questions of why one woman will fall victim to endometriosis and not another: Is the susceptibility traceable to a balance or imbalance, of some combination of factors? Can you accidentally give yourself endometriosis as a result of a fall or any other accident? How implicated are birth control pills or even intrauterine influences from before you were born? You cannot know if you are having this particular disorder or not because the symptoms of this disease are extremely common and natural. One may ignore them too but the effects are extremely troubling. Could it get any worse when you'll get to know you cannot conceive? Yes, infertility is one of its adverse effects. So it's better to look into the symptoms and get started with the treatment in the shortest of time before it gets too late. Its major symptoms are as below;

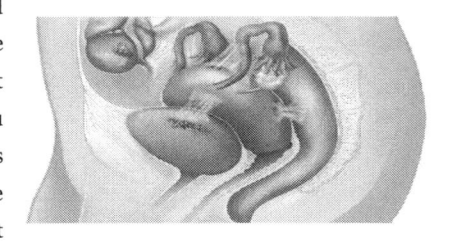

- **Painful periods:** Pelvic pain is natural and pretty ordinary during periods but the pain during endometriosis is slightly different as begins almost 5-7 days before and extends several days into your period and may include lower back and abdominal pain also.
- **Excessive bleeding:** You may experience an occasional heavy bleeding (menorrhagia) or un occasional bleeding between the periods (Menometrorrhagia)
- **Pain during sex:** Painful intercourse is another serious problem of endometriosis victims. Endometrial lesions, especially when they are trapped and growing in the cul-de-sac can push the uterus into an

extroverted position. Retroversion is a tilting back of the uterus. When the uterus is thus pulled out of its normal position, deep vaginal penetration during intercourse can be extremely painful.
- **RECTAL BLEEDING:** blood in the urine or the need to urinate frequently during menstruation can also indicate endometriosis. And if a woman feels pain radiating from her buttocks to the outside of her legs, her sciatic nerve may be affected.
- **INFERTILITY:** women are unable to get pregnant due to this disorder. It is first diagnosed in the women who seeking treatment to conceive.
- **OTHER SYMPTOMS:** Diarrhea, nausea, constipation, pain with bowel movements and fatigue during periods especially are most likely to be experienced too.

CAUSES OF ENDOMETRIOSIS

- Although the actual causes of this disorder have yet not found out but some assumed causes include;
- Attachment to surgical incision: after a surgery or C section, endometrial cells may attach to a surgical incision which causes the endometriosis.
- Embryonic cell growth: Embryonic cells are the cells that make the pelvic and abdominal lining. So when small areas convert into the endometrial tissue, endometriosis can develop.
- Reversed menstruation: This is one of the most accepted causes. When the menstrual blood flows back in the fallopian tubes instead of out of the body, these cells stick to the pelvic walls where they grow and cause the bleeding of each menstrual cycle.
- Other causes: An immune system disorder could also be one of the causes where the body is unable to recognize and destroy the endometrial cells outside the uterus. The endometrial cells transport could also be one of the causes.

THE AFFECTED AREAS:

Most often the ovaries, fallopian tubes, and tissue around the uterus are affected, however, in some rare cases it may also occur in some other part of the body but basically these three parts are the affected parts of the body which are also quite sensitive.

OVARIAN CANCER: The highest rate of ovarian cancer occurring is in the women with endometriosis. Some studies suggest that endometriosis increases the risk but it is still relatively low and not that common. Another rare type of cancer – endometriosis-associated-adenocarcinoma – can also develop in the women.

CHAPTER TWO HOW TO PREVENT ENDOMETRIOSIS

The removal of endometriosis is a basic demand for most of the women. But majority wants to get rid of it so they can conceive and get pregnant. If you truly want to get over this disease, you definitely can. Just remain persistent and don't give up thinking it cannot get cured. There may be a few successes for those who choose conventional drugs and surgery to treat this disorder, but they are few and far between. The best long term success tends to be for those who use natural and alternative methods to treat endometriosis. This is because using natural therapies are natural. They cure the disease with the help of your own immune system without damaging any other part of your body. And since healing comes from within so the alternative therapies also strengthen your immune system to work appropriately. Such therapies are also permanent and not temporary.

NATURAL THERAPIES:

DIETARY CHANGES
- Eat as much organic food as you can and avoid and factory farmed meats because they contain the growth hormones which is not good. Iron must be taken regularly.
- Avoid white flour and white rice because they contain some traces of dioxins which are always a byproduct of chlorine.
- Honey is appreciated too as it is an anti-inflammatory sweetener.
- Use non-homogenized milk instead of homogenized milk.
- Avoid soy products and intake of processed foods.

CASTOR OIL RECOMMENDATION
When you initially start getting cramps, a castor oil transdermal pack can be used to reduce the severity of the symptoms. Soak a washed cloth in pure castor oil and put it the bare skin on the lower stomach. Then place a hot water bottle on top of that and leave for 30 minutes at least and you'll feel a noticeable change.

USE OF COMBINED CONTRACEPTIVES:

The combined oral contraceptive pill is not just one drug. Rather, there are many different types, each of which contains a specific low-dose combination of synthetic estrogen and progestin (progesterone).The main advantages of the pill are that it is inexpensive and is usually reasonably well tolerated by women. These drugs do not eliminate endometriosis but alleviates the pain by suppressing menstruation and inhibiting the growth of the endometrial implants.

Exercise: It is the best way to kick endometriosis. Sweating is the only way to cleanse the lymph nodes, and endometriosis is a disease that is influenced by toxicity so exercising a week before the menstrual cycle can be very beneficial.

Usage of birth control pills: Usage of birth control pills may stop the menstrual period altogether, which can reduce or eliminate the pain. So it is one temporary solution.

Intake of naproxen: There are many drugs which could be taken for killing the pain. This is not a permanent solution for endometriosis but acts as an anti-inflammatory painkiller.

Surgical removal: The surgery will help the removal of the endometrial tissue to improve the fertility. There are three kinds of surgeries;

- laparoscopy (the most commonly used and least invasive technique)
- laparotomy
- hysterectomy

Laparoscopy is the most common technique where the surgeon inserts an instrument and removes an endometriosis cyst which is growing on an ovary whereas laparotomy is a key whole surgery where the surgeons see the extent of endometriosis around the uterus. And hysterectomy is for those who don't plan on getting pregnant as it helps in the removal of the ovaries.

HORMONAL THERAPY: Supplemental hormones are sometimes used to eliminate the pain of endometriosis. The hormonal therapy causes the slowdown of the growth of endometrial tissues and prevents new implants of it. But it is no way a permanent solution for endometriosis.

- Gonadotropin-releasing hormone: This drug helps to prevent menstruation by blocking the production of ovarian-stimulating hormones and lowering the estrogen level which causes the endometrial tissues to shrink. Since they create an artificial menopause so they also result in decreasing the side effects such as hot flashes, vaginal dryness and bone loss.
- Danazol: This is slightly dangerous as is has side effects and is often now recommended. It can be harmful to the baby if you become pregnant while taking this medicine. But its main function is to block the production of ovarian-stimulating hormone and prevent menstruation.

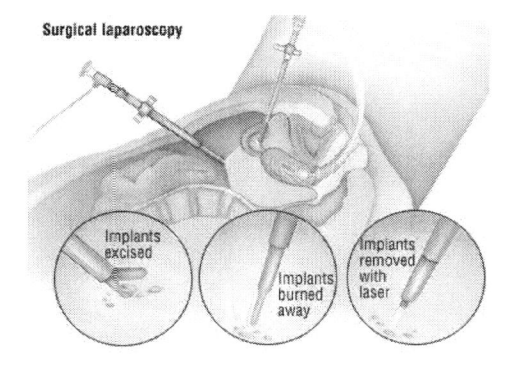

Surgical laparoscopy

Chapter Three Health Recipes to Prevent Endometriosis

'He who takes medicine and neglects to diet wastes the skill of his doctors'- Chinese proverb.

An appropriate diet for any kind of disease is as important as the medicines are, so it shall be given equal importance and must not be neglected in any case. In order to regenerate your health by reducing the symptoms of endometriosis, the change in your diet is significant.

Adjusting what you eat can bring many conclusive physical changes by reducing symptoms of pain, relieving cramps, reducing inflammation, reducing bloating and estrogen levels, balancing hormones, or precisely by increasing energy levels and improving overall health. Similarly, endometriosis is no exception in responding positively to the diet changes.

Here are some recipes that can help you to improve your health while suffering from endometriosis as they are Vegan, Gluten free, wheat free, soya free, refined sugar free, rice free and endometriosis safe.

Chocolate cheesecake

Ingredients:
- 4oz Raw Cashew Nuts
- 3.5oz Honey
- 2.5oz Cocoa Powder
- 2 Tsp. vanilla Paste
- 2oz Coconut Oil
- 1oz Pure Spread
- Half an Avocado

Crust:

- 2oz Almond Butter
- 3oz Dates
- 1oz Coconut Oil
- 1 Tsp. Vanilla Paste
- 2 Tsp. Hazelnut milk

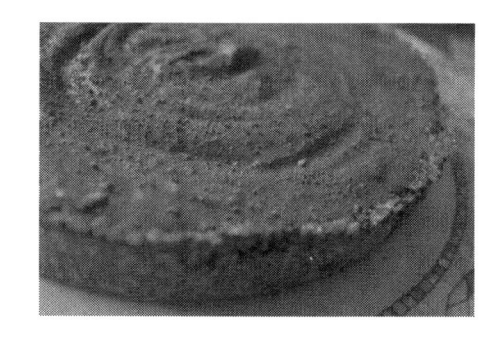

Method:
1) Soak the cashew nuts for two hours to make them soft.
2) Line your cake tin with a baking paper.
3) Put all the ingredients into a high speed blender until turn thick and stick together easily.
4) Take some of your mixture and press it firmly into the bottom of your mold in order to make the first layer of your cake.
5) To make a cheesecake, put the soaked and drained cashew nuts into the blender along with the agave nectar and put the blender on high until you have a smooth nut mixture.
6) Then add the cocoa powder and put the blender on low and build it up to medium eventually.
7) Melt the pure coconut oil and pour it in the blender along with the mixture and keep blending on medium them high.
8) In the appeared paste, now add half of an avocado and blend for a minute or two and a smooth chocolate will appear.
9) Spoon the mixture on the top of the crust into your cake tin and put them into the fridge for a couple of hours and then take it out of the mould and peel away the baking paper and enjoy your cheesecake.

HOT CHOCOLATE

INGREDIENTS:
Left over mixture of the chocolate cheesecake
250 ml Hazelnut Milk

METHOD:
1) Instead of washing your blender after making the chocolate cheesecake's mixture, pour milk and blend it for 5 minutes.
2) Your chocolate milk is now absolutely ready to serve. So place it in a glass and garnish some chocolate over it to give it a better look.

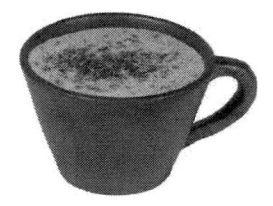

Scrumptious Halibut Pasta

Ingredients:
- Handful of 100% Corn Pasta
- 1 Piece of frozen/fresh Halibut fish
- Peas
- Chestnuts
- 1 Tsp. Fine Herbs
- Drizzle of Extra Virgin Olive Oil

Sauce:
- 2 Tsp. Extra Virgin Olive Oil
- 1 Tsp. Vinegar
- 2 Tsp. Bouillon Vegan Stock
- ½ Tsp. Mustard Sauce

Method:

1) Place your Halibut Fish into a piece of foil and drizzle extra virgin olive oil on it. Then sprinkle your fine herbs onto the fish and wrap it up into a foil paper before you put it onto a tray and cook it for 5-20 minutes in the oven.

2) While the fish is cooking, boil the peas and chestnuts and also boil the pasta until becomes soft.

3) Then mix all the sauce ingredients well and pour it into the pasta whose water was drained off and mix the peas and chestnuts in it as well.

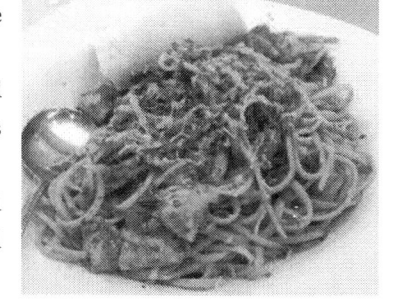

4) Till all this procedure, the fish must have got cooked so unwrap the foil carefully, scoop out the fish and pop it on the pasta.

5) Now mash up the fish into chunks with your fork and sprinkle natural yeast flakes on it if you want to.

SNOWBALL TRUFFLES

INGREDIENTS:
- 2oz Almond Butter
- 3oz Dates
- 1oz Coconut Flour + Some for rolling
- 1 Tsp. Vanilla Extract
- 2 Tsp. Hazelnut Milk

METHOD:
- Put all the ingredients into the blender and blend them from low to medium gradually.
- A sticky mixture will be obtained which should be roll into little balls.
- Then dip those balls into the coconut flour and apply a little pressure so the flour sticks to it properly.

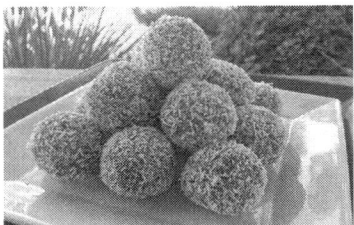

Brusque Mixed Herb Bread

INGREDIENTS:
- 3.5oz Almond Flour
- 3.5oz Sorghum Flour
- 2oz Sogo Powder
- 2oz Potato Flour
- 2oz Arrowroot Powder
- 1 Tsp. Xanthan gum
- 2 Tsp. unrefined sugar
- 1 Tsp. baking powder
- 1 Tsp. Coconut Oil
- 3 Heaped Tsp. Bart's Fine/ Mixed Herbs
- 215ml Warm Water

METHOD:
1) Preheat the oven gas mark 6/ 200 degree Celsius
2) Combine unrefined sugar, xanthium gum, salt and baking powder in a bowl together.
3) Next add the arrowroot powder, Sago powder, Almond flour and potato flour together with mixed herbs and mix together.
4) Melt the coconut oil with ladle over a naked flame and add the melted coconut oil to the mixture and stir it.
5) Add the warm water slowly as you go and you dough looks soft and smooth. And if it looks dry, then add a little water to it.
6) The dough isn't elastic because there is no gluten added to it so to knead the dough, pick it up and squish it altogether so everything could be mixed properly.
7) Roll the dough and keep kneading the mixture for a couple of minutes.

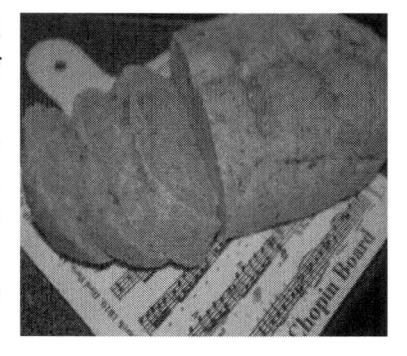

8) Cover with foil, put it onto a tray and into the pre-heated over for 40-45 minutes and then for last 5-10 minutes take the foil off until turns brown and golden.
9) Leave it to cool down a little and eat it the same day it's been cooked.

Apricot and Chocolate Mousse

Ingredients:
- 4oz Cashews
- 3oz Agave Nectar
- 4 Tbs. Almond Milk
- 3oz Carob
- 1 Tsp. Vanilla Paste
- 2oz Cocoa butter
- 1oz Pure Spread
- 1oz Water
- 8 Apricots

Method:
1) Soak the cashews in boiling water for 2 hours.
2) Melt the cocoa butter and put 4oz Cashews, 3oz Agave Nectar, 4 Tbs. Almond Milk, 3oz Carob, 1 Tsp. Vanilla Paste, 2oz Cocoa butter, 1oz Pure Spread, 1oz Water into a blender and blend until nice and smooth.
3) Next add the apricots and continue blending until they are finely chopped.
4) On obtaining a lumpy mixture, add carob and blend it again in the addition of some water.
5) Blend a little longer so it gets lighter to have a moose texture/
6) Now scoop it in a bowl and put it in the refrigerator.

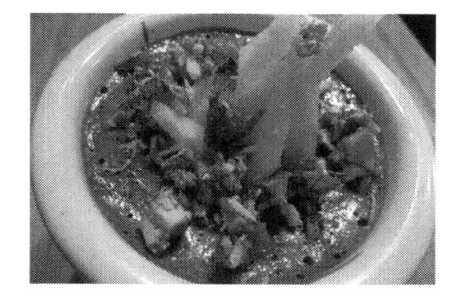

Pie Pastry

Ingredients:
- 1 3/4oz Millet Flour
- 1 3/4oz Quinoa Flour
- 1 3/4oz Gluten Free Oat Flour
- 3oz Almond Flour
- 2 Tbs. Potato Starch
- 2 Tbs. Arrowroot Powder
- 1 Tsp. Xanthan Gum
- 4oz Pure Spread
- 1 Baking Powder
- 3 Tsp. Ground Flax Seed
- 6 Tsp. Hot Water
- 5 Tbs. Hot Water
- 1oz Sorghum Flour

Method:
1) Mix the ground flax seeds with hot water and leave on the side to turn gloopy.
2) Add all of the dry ingredients into a bowl with the pure spread and rub it into the flour. It should form a loose ball.
3) Now add the flax and combine all the materials.
4) In a separate bowl, mix the sorghum flour and warm water until a paste is formed.
5) Now add the sorghum mix into the pastry. Fold the dough a few times and your pie pastry is ready. It could be enjoyable when baked.

Ambrosial vegetable pie

Ingredients:
- 1 Courgette
- ½ Onion
- 3 Asparagus Stalks
- ½ of a Leek
- 3 Mushrooms
- 2 Tsp. Natural Yeast Flakes
- Drizzle of Extra Virgin Olive Oil

Method:
1) First, make a pastry according to the previous recipe and fill it in a metal pie by chopping off the edges for a nice clean look.
2) Line the pie with baking paper and fill them with clay bead to blind bake the pastry.
3) Then put them in the oven on gas mark 5 for 23-30 minutes until turn lovely golden color.
4) Now paint the inside of the pastry with the homemade pesto (recipe given). With the back of a spoon, spread the pesto right up to the top of your pastry cases.
5) Now chop the cougette and layer the pieces to line the bottom of the pie.
6) Next chop the onions and asparagus stalks and layers those on the top of courgettes.
7) Chop the leek and mushroom and layer those on top also. This finish off the pie with a little natural yeast flakes being dusted upon.
8) By drizzling extra virgin olive oil over the top, put it into the already preheated oven for 15-20 minutes and serve it with mash potatoes or potato salad.

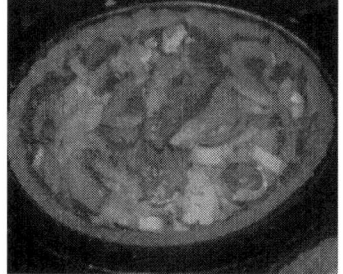

Double Chocolate Mud Pies

Ingredients:
- ½ of the Pie Pastry (recipe mentioned above)
- Mousse Filling (recipe mentioned above)
- Just miss the apricots or keep them in, they are lovely either way

Double chocolate:
2oz Carob

Method:
1) Squish the pastry into the cake tins and prick the bottom of the pastry cases with a fork.
2) Do the same if you are making double chocolate mud pies. Also prick the bottom.
3) Pop them into the oven on gas mark 5 for 20-25 minutes.
4) Once turn golden, take them out and wait for the cases to cool before adding chocolate mousse.
5) By adding sprinkle of carob to the top of the pies, enjoy the firm but light pies.

Presto Pesto

Ingredients:
- 2 Big Handfuls of Spinach
- 2 Big Handfuls of Kale
- 2 Cloves of Garlic
- 1.5oz Almond Flour
- 2 Tbs. Natural Yeast Flakes
- 60ml Extra Virgin Olive Oil (Add more if you like it loose)
- Pinch of Salt & Pepper

Method:
1) Add all the ingredients to a blender and blend until a lovely thick sauce is formed.
2) If you don't like thick then add as much water as you want to, to get your personal perfect consistency.
3) Put the paste into some jar; keep it in fridge and use in different recipes too.
4) If the pesto becomes a little thicker then add one or two drops of extra virgin olive oil to get it back to its original shape.

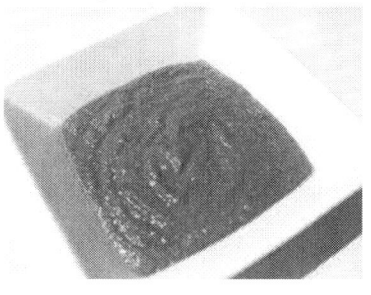

Two nut free caramels

Ingredients:
- 2.5oz any Seed Butter
- 4 Tbs. Agave nectar
- 5 heaped Tbs. unrefined Light Brown Sugar
- 1 Tsp. Vanilla Paste
- 2 Tbs. Pure Spread

Chocolate:
3 heaped tsp. Carob Powder

Method:
1) Add all the ingredients to a blender and blend until turn into a smooth mixture.
2) Take out the caramel mixture and put it into a pan on a low-medium heat.
3) Keep stirring until the caramel is sticky and pulling together nicely.
4) Place the caramel mixture into a piece of baking paper and form into the desired shape. Wrap it up and put it in the freezer.
5) After about 25 minutes the caramel will be hard and ready for munching.

Chocolate Caramels

Method:
1) Follow the above recipe but add cocoa powder also and blend it altogether.
2) Add the mixture to a pan on low-medium heat and keep stirring.
3) The mixture will melt and again thicken up due to the pure and sugar.
4) Place the caramel onto a piece of baking paper and form into your desired shape.
5) Wrap up the caramel and stick it in to the freezer for 25 minutes till become hard.

Chapter Four Tips for happiness and productivity

Who on earth doesn't want to be happy? Doesn't want to kick depression and distress? But the question is whether happiness really is a priority for you at this point in time? Are you really doing you maximum to live a happy life? Could you be doing any more to live a happy and fulfilling life? If you think you could make some improvement in making yourself happy then there is undoubtedly a lot to come.

What actually is happiness? Everyone has their own definition and gets happy over various things but for me happiness is something that encompasses the entire positive from what I call the "low arousal" ones such as contentment, calm and satisfaction, through to the "high arousal" ones such as joy and excitement. You need to become an "extrovert" to seek out and experience more of the high arousal positive emotions in order to live an excited and relaxed life.

There are infinite ways to get happier but you just have to be determined on the strategies which are important to you and make sure you dedicate time on regular basis to master the relevant skills.

Don't tolerate negative thoughts: Do you know what is the biggest enemy to your happiness? Unhelpful and self-defeating thoughts! Make sure you learn to control you mind and especially, how to identify and challenge the pessimistic thoughts.

Live in the moment: Don't ever think happiness will come in the future or you've had enough of happiness in your life. No. You can make every moment precious if you want to. Happy people spend less time dwelling on the past, and worrying about the future, and more time living in the here and now.

ENJOY EVERY BIT OF YOUR LIFE: Now there is a difference between living the moment and enjoying it thoroughly. Happy people are more thankful, they are grateful on what they have and think less about what they don't. They notice small things that others don't ever care for. Sometimes they are happy just because!

FOCUS ON THE STRENGTHS YOU HAVE: Everyone knows how to fix their weaknesses but what I love the most about happy people is that they know how to utilize their core strengths, qualities and attributes. So just focus on the things you're good at and find ways to do more of those as often as possible.

GET TO KNOW YOURSELF: Imagine yourself walking down the street with each one of your values. How do you feel? What do you notice? How are you expressing yourself? This will help you identify yourself through your own eyes instead of through the eyes of others. Try to know who you are? What things do you want from life? What are your need and demands? And everything affiliated to you and your soul.

TAKE CARE OF YOUR NEEDS: According to us the best way of becoming happy is by making the other person happy through fulfilling their need but that causes us to live our lives through the eyes of others and not from our core. Instead of this, just think of the things that could make YOU happy. Start practicing at least one thing each day that gives you comfort and ease.

MEDITATE: Meditation is one of the most important things to lead a calm life. We are all the time busy thinking something and our brain never gets rest but in meditation you have to calm your mind by connecting to your deepest self. And this is how we can unfold the mystery of our own happiness.

WORK WITH YOUR FEARS: we all have some fears that we are drenched into. Learn to get rid of them by having a staunch control over them. When you repress and reject your fears because of unrealistic expectations of being perfect that society imposes on us, you will be granting more power and control to your fears.

LET GO OF THE PAST: Do not ruin your present over past. Don't let the past haunt you and inflict more suffering in your life rather just learn to forgive yourself and move ahead. There is so much more waiting for you because when one door closes, many others open up so cheers.

SMILE: The best you can do to yourself is SMILE. It is contagious. If you are feeling down in the dumps, force to smile and keep smiling. It will give you a sort of inner satisfaction and will genuinely make you feel good. Try it once.

DO LESS: It is a tip for both, happiness as well as productivity. Doing less will give you time for your loved ones, for the things that give you pleasure and for life itself. It will exempt you from the stress and hectic routine. Focus on the big, essential tasks of your life and eliminate the rest, you will actually be more productive that way. No matter, the number of tasks will be fewer but they will satisfy you at least.

SLOW DOWN: Your life will be more pleasurable when you slow down the things. You will learn and enjoy much more once you start doing your think slowly and with full concentration. Slowing down things give you so much relaxation like drive slower, walk slower, eat slower, talk slower etc.

GET ORGANIZED: People enjoy being messy but try being organized once. It feels amazing. You find yourself extremely focused once things get organized. It is so much enjoyable too.

SIMPLIFY YOUR FINANCES: Want to reduce your stress? Cut down your finances. Reduce the number of bank accounts, credit cards, spend less and reduce your bills. Make your finances auto magical and you will feel extremely quenched.

DO NOT COMPARE YOURSELF TO OTHERS: Accept what you are and what you have. I know it's difficult but whenever you start comparing yourself to others, a friend, co-worker, a model etc. just stop. And think you are different. With different struggles and different aims in life and start counting your qualities and blessings that you've been bestowed upon.

LEARN TO LOSE ARGUMENTS: This is especially for the married people. Seek to understand instead of giving up or trying to win on every argument. Learn to understand the other person's point of view from their position rather than fighting over and not getting quiet.

ENJOY THE LITTLE THINGS: Big things certainly bring you big pleasure but your life will be heaven if you start noticing and enjoying small things that come in your life. You will feel blessed literally. Stop and notice what you are doing right now and look around. And take time to enjoy it.

Chapter Five WHY do people gain weight?

Obesity is an excess of body fat in relation to muscle and other lean tissues. Obesity reflex a long term imbalance in the amount of calories consumed in the diet and the amount of calories used in physical activity and maintenance of body processes. Development of obesity, however, is more complicated than just calories in vs. calories out. It is a complex issue and is caused by a combination of physiological, psychological, and so sociological factors that begin in childhood and are reinforced throughout life.

Obesity can be divided into two categories: obesity caused by an excess consumption of calories and obesity caused by an internal imbalance. As evidence accumulates it might be accepted that most cases of obesity are a result of internal imbalance and that calorie consumption is secondary to these imbalances. This doesn't mean that obesity is incurable. It does mean that an overweight person who eats a little food and struggles to lose weight should not feel guilty or ashamed for "lack of willpower". Regardless of the origin of obesity, there are guidelines to lose access weight and maintain weight loss.

THE GENETICS THEORY: a tendency to gain access weight might be inherited.

Children of obese parents have a greater likelihood of becoming over weight than do children of normal weight parents.

Studies on identical and non-identical twins show that weight gain might be result of genetic factors. The genetic influences on weight gain are more likely to occur in a person who is overweight from childhood.

THE ENVIRONMENT THEORY:

The most popular theory of obesity states they being overweight are a result of the environment. A person may consume more calories by the following ways:
- the behavior was learned from the parents;
- a person overreacts to outside cues such as television commercials;
- a person lacks discipline or "will power".

The environment theory states that behavior is learned and that eating patterns promote weigh gain are reinforced by environmental cues and pressures. The behavior modification approach to a weight control is based on this theory.

THE FAT CELL THEORY: The number of fat cells KN the body might result from over eating early in life rather than genetics. Fat tissue can expand in two ways: an increase in thru number of fat cells or an increase in the size of fat cells.

During infancy, childhood, adolescence and pregnancy, growth is rapid and both the number and size of cells increase. Once the fat cells are formed they are not destroyed, but their size can increase or decrease with growing age.

Weight loss can reduce the size of the fat cell but not the number of cells. The overfed child or adolescent has more fat cells and a greater tendency for obesity later in life.

THE BROWN FAT THEORY: most calories from the diet are used to maintain body functions such as hair growth, breathing and digestion. Another portion of the daily calorie intake is used to fuel physical activity such as walking, shopping or cooking. Some calories are used to produce heat, a process that includes a specific type of fat called brown fat.

The loss of energy or heat after eating is called "diet-induced thermo genesis." The brown fat or diet induced thermo genie response to eating might explain why some people can overeat and not gain weight while others cannot. In addition, the amount of heat loss is related to the total surface area of the body. A tall heavy person has more surface area than a short light one.

THE ENZYME THEORY: enzymes are protein like substances in the body that regulate all chemical reactions. For example, enzymes dissolve food during digestion, facilitate the formation of protein and all substances in the cell and convert carbohydrates to energy. Obese people might use blood sugar for energy, rather than a mixture of sugar and fat. When sugar stores are used, the obese person experiences low blood sugar and is hungry more often than the learner person who burns a combination of fat and sugar.

THE SET POINT THE THEORY: The set point theory states that living organisms have a predetermined fat reserve that will be defended no matter what the challenge. For example animals are starved to the point of obesity, return to their previous fat storage level and normal weight when allowed to regulate their own diets.

This set point for body fat might be found in humans and would account for some people to lose weight, but not maintain the weight loss. The body loses weight in the starvation or dieting period and gains back the fat stores in an effort to return to what the body considers normal.

Some people might have an abnormally high set point that interferes with permanent weight loss. Whereas the restriction of calories apparent cannot overcome a high set point, physical activity, especially aerobic exercise, might lower a person's set point and provide the means for permanent weight loss.

CARBOHYDRATE BALANCE THEORIES: Carbohydrates have been promoted as high calories food that encourages weight gain. This is not true for all carbohydrates. The dietary recommendations for people to reduce the incidence of obesity, cardiovascular disease, diabetes, hypertension and cancer suggest an increase in the consumption of complex carbohydrates.

Carbohydrate foods are divided into two categories: sugar and starch. Foods high in simple carbohydrates include syrup, pie and sweets. Complex carbohydrate foods are rice, pasta, whole grain and refined grain products, dried beans and peas and starchy vegetables. Carbohydrates provide a readily available source of energy to the body.

The carbohydrate theory of weight control states the appetite center in the hypothalamus and specialized cells in the liver and sensitive to the level of glucose in the blood.

A diet high in sugar might upset appetite regulation. When blood sugar levels are elevated, the appetite center and specialized liver cells signal the brain that the person is full and the person stops eating. When levels are low, messages are sent to the brain that it is time to eat.

This theory might explain why some people overeat. Appetite and hunger might be a result of carbohydrates content of the diet. After food is eaten, the hormone insulin is released to help transport the blood sugar glucose into the cells for nourishments. The amount of insulin released is related to the amount of carbohydrate, the greater the amount of insulin released. When blood sugar is normal, a person feels satisfied. When blood sugar drops, a person feels hungry.

Hunger increases as the insulin transports the sugar out of blood and into the cells. This process is exaggerated when the dietary carbohydrate is sugar. A person might feel weak, anxious, or uneasy because of low blood sugar. Soon after the ingestion of a sugary food such as a chocolate bar, a person might feel better. The feelings of hunger and weakness return, however, within an hour or two when the simple sugar has been absorbed, digested, and removed by the insulin from blood.

Complex carbohydrates and starch are digested and absorbed slowly. They do not cause the rapid rise in blood sugar that is seen with sugar and so do not trigger excess insulin secretion and the drop in blood sugar.

Some people might be "carbohydrate cravers" because of the calming effects or drowsiness, these people experience after eating a meal high in carbohydrates. This relaxation might be a result of the effects of insulin or insulin and serotonin.

Serotonin is a hormone like compound in the brain from the amino acid tryptophan. Serotonin regulates mood, sleep, pain, and other behaviors. Tryptophan must cross the lining of the intestine and then travel to the brain before it is available for conversion to serotonin.

Tryptophan competes with other amino acids for entry into the brain. If a person consumes a high protein meal only moderate amounts of these amino acids enter the brain. A high carbohydrates/ low protein meals help remove amino acids that compete with tryptophan for entry into the brain: more tryptophan enters the brain and the synthesis of the serotonin in the brain increases. This might improve sleep and cause the drowsiness reported by some people after a carbohydrate meal.

If a person is a carbohydrate craver, he or she might want to include enough complex carbohydrate in a diet to main the level of comfort.

CHAPTER SIX HOW TO LOSE WEIGHT?

Quick weigh loss diets are popular for several reasons:
- People want to believe the diet will work. Losing and maintaining weight is not easy. People become discouraged by the failure of other more traditional methods of weight loss and are willing to try anything.
- It is human nature to look for the easy way out for a problem, to want something for nothing, and to avoid the effort, frustration, the risk of failure that is essential to success.

Table 1 Myths About Weight Loss
In addition to the fad diets, a person must be alert to the fallacies that surround weigh reduction. These are commonly held fallacies related to weight control:
1. Obesity is entirely due to heredity.
2. In the experience id some people, all foods turn to fat.
3. Make slipping is a good way to lose weight.
4. You can eat all you want and still reduce weight by taking the reducing pills.
5. Special low calorie bread should be used in reducing weight.
6. Toast has fewer calories than bread.
7. One must not drink water while trying for weight loss.
8. Sweets enriched with vitamins maybe eaten when a person is reducing.
9. Washing rice after cooking reduces weight.
10. Sugar is not as fattening as starch.
11. High protein foods and fruits have no calories.
12. Jelly dessert is nonfattening.
13. Milk should not be included in a weight reduction diet.
14. Meat burns its own calories.
15. Margarine contains fewer calories than butter.

> 16. For reducing, eat high protein goods for a week; then eat anything you want for a week.

There is hardly any person on this planet who doesn't want to lose weight and get smart. It's more like a battle that's been fought across the globe by almost everyone. But weight loss is just not physical but also a mental activity.

The first step to lose weight and keep it off permanently is to make a commitment, not to anyone else but your own and then get determined on it. You are losing weight because YOU want to, not to keep others happy. You just have to become internally motivated because that is what will pump you the most towards your goal. Find a particular routine that fix to your lifestyle and then get stick to it. So precisely, stop pleasing others and become self-motivated

The second step is to devote you completely and follow all the steps that are required. Losing weight naturally helps us to live a way better and healthier lifestyle that can eventually boost our confidence. And continuing to live like this helps us to prolong our lives.

Food containing important nutrients can help us prevent diseases and even restore our health. Striking a balance between healthy eating and foods that may be risky is important for long term wellbeing. Choose foods that are better for your health more often. Without a doubt, fats and cholesterol are the single most important group of nutrients to limit when healthy eating is the goal and if you want to reduce your risk of chronic disease. Heart disease and cancer, two of the nation's leading killers, are linked to diets high in fat.

There are many ways to lose weight some of the most effective methods that can help you lose weight really fast and without any pain are as following;

EAT HEALTHY: The best way to lose weight is not to starve you but just eat the right proportion of healthy food. Stay away from fried things and especially the ones that contain bulk of fats. Carbohydrates should be kept at minimum too. All they do is provide bulk which is extremely difficult to break down. So eat fresh fruits, vegetables, milk, meat, proteins and juices in an appropriate proportion

EXERCISE: Eating healthy just keeps you from getting fat but exercise is what keeps you lose your weight. For example in order to reduce the fats from thighs, lunges and squats are the two perfect ways. Similarly two set of ten sit ups or crunches will help you lose your fats from the stomach area. Exercise also tones up your body muscles and keeps body active.

DRINK WATER: Water is the basic necessity of life. Drink as much water as you can but eight glasses of water is a normal ratio in a day. Avoid drinking sugary, alcoholic or fizzy drinks as it contains carbohydrates.

SLEEP: Take at least eight to ten hours of sleep as it won't make you feel any lethargic and you would feel fresh instead. Your body also build muscles while you snooze, getting zzz's equals better muscle tone.

WAIT UNTIL YOUR STOMACH RUMBLES BEFORE YOU REACH THE FOOD: More than hunger, we eat food due to boredom, nervousness, habit or just frustration forgetting what physical hunger actually feels like. If you badly want any particular food, then it's craving not hunger. Try to eat only in that condition when you are finding "anything" to eat. That is the time when you are genuinely hungry.

EAT IN FRONT OF MIRRORS: Eating in front of mirror can help you lose weight as it reminds you of your inner standards and goals and makes you recall why you're trying to lose weight in the first place.

WALK: Walk minimum five minutes for at least every two hours. It will make you less likely to reach for snacks out of antsiness and will help you make less lazy. If you walk for

45 minutes a day, it can help you lose 30 pounds in a year regardless of how much you eat the entire years. But it should be a brisk walk.

ORDER THE SMALLEST PORTION OF EVERYTHING: Never give up eating by killing yourself from the inside. You can definitely crave for anything at any time so it's better to order the smallest portion of it. If you want popcorns, get the smallest pack, small drink, small salad etc. If we would get ourselves the maximum size, we'd eat if unintentionally and unwillingly so better keep the minimum to yourself.

EAT MINIMUM IN YOUR DINNER: This tip is just not for the ones who are dieting but for everyone. Heavy dinner make you bulky and fat over a short time period. Because instantly after dinner, you get to sleep which doesn't burn off any calories instead it gets stored and makes you healthy.

Chapter seven Simplification in Life

Everyone has a different meaning for simple life but for me, it means to kick out all the stress by making things less complicated. One major step which can help you lead a simple life is; identify what is important to you and eliminate everything else from your life. This doesn't mean to ignore the things that make you happy, no. But just disregard certain things to be left with the things we value and love.

"Nothing is enough for the man to whom enough is too little." We have made our lives so much complicated and fussy over no big reasons at all. It's just our minds and not the things that is the reason behind. This is usually due to the absence of an important thing in life which makes us so worried and chaotic. So what it all requires is to have a work-life balance. We must give equal time to work, family, a lover, friends, leisure pursuits and spirituality.

Why simplification in life is important? It helps us to live a life in peace and not chaos, a life of essentials and not complications and a life of needs and not wants. We will slow down and stop living the frazzled life, a lifestyle of stress. We will learn to relax in the limited resources we have with us. We will live a good life of pleasure, flow, meaning and purpose with private time and solitude.

Nothing in this life is permanent, so be happy with what you have and cherish the moments you are spending right now. Everything changes so let's focus on our time, energy and financial resources and not wait for a crisis. Let's eliminate clutter, which distracts us from the important things in life. Learn to live your life within your means and avoid the burden of a mountain of debt. This will help you live your life mindfully, in the present moment, and not ruminate with worry of the future or regrets of past. "If you ask what the single most important key to longevity is, I would have to say it is avoiding worry, stress and tension. And if you didn't ask me, I'd still have to say it." –

George F. Burns

It is not an easy thing to be done but it is not impossible either. You have to ignore what has packed on stress in your life while still being able to maintain the activities that are important to you. Get over the luxuries in your life which gives you no good and make your life simple. Things that don't relax you and yet you are continuing them, LEAVE them.

Limit YOU'RE communications: Our life these days are filled with vast flow of communications: email, cell phones, Skype, twitter, Facebook, forums and much more. You can spend your entire day on these things. Instead, put a limit on your communications: use all these things for a particular time period when important. Set a schedule and stick to it.

Acceptance of what you have: To stay happy and contended to have to accept the things you have and become thankful for them. You have been blessed with such a pleasant life. You are better from so many other people around, physically as well as financially. And your life will become even better when you start accepting the things you have and be happy with them. Instead of looking at the people who are leading a luxurious life than you, look at those who are living their lives in a misery. Who can't even afford to eat or sleep? Who doesn't have a shelter of their own? You are better than so many people. So why not be thankful for the things you already have?

Complain less: Currently, the biggest complain I hear is about the price of petrol. You certainly cannot control the price of petrol but you can control its usage. So instead of complaining about everything every time, look for another way out that could be helpful. The appreciation for everything leads you to increased personal power.

LEARN TO SAY NO: Saying no to inappropriate things can help you increase your self-esteem, self-respect and more time to what you love. It is not necessary to say yes to everything because you don't owe anyone a reason or an excuse. If the person persists, say no to him again, the person will eventually get your message.

DON'T MEDDLE IN OTHER PEOPLE'S BUSINESS. Concentrate on keeping your own life in order, and don't worry about everyone else's.

ENJOY WITHOUT OWNING. Admire the objects in a shop window, the art in a gallery, the plants in a garden, without acquiring them for yourself. You'll often get more

CHAPTER EIGHT A GOAL IN LIFE

You can do nothing without setting certain goals in your life. Having a goal written down for accomplishment gives you something to plan and work for. Makes you active and represents you inner desires. It's a constant reminder of what and when you need to accomplish. There is a common pattern to that comes with setting a goal: you set your mind to something, you get excited and work like crazy, and then motivation starts to wane. Goals give you inner desires and energy to work on them throughout the period.

When you see a massive, insurmountable mountain, it seems impossible to climb for you. But proper goal setting can help break larger, intimidating aspirations into smaller, more achievable stepping stones. Planning to accomplish such bigger goals help you formulate a definite plan of action that we can start working on right now. The best way to climb such a mountain is by splitting it into smaller hills in your own mind. You'll be happier and motivated with every hill climbing by.

Setting goals for yourself is a way to fuel your ambitions. It gives us an inspiration necessary to aim for things we never thought possible rather than just creating a plan and holding accountable. Try to make slow and steady progress by every day passing by because if there is not progress in achieving, you dreams and aspirations are nothing more than vague notions floating around in your imagination.

While achieving a goal, there comes a time when we think we really don't need what we ever planned for. We don't need this much money, when really we need a change in our life or someone we love whom we could see happy by spending our money over. Sometimes we think we need some free time, when really we want is work that we can truly feel passionate about. Sometime we want to be alone but we actually need some positive or happy people around. By asking ourselves what we really want and constantly re-assessing our goals, we gain the benefit of self-reflection. We get to figure out the actual thing we have been looking for in life – and then we can go out and do it.

Whenever you set any goal in life just make sure you get the maximum out of every moment. Don't hesitate in experiencing something new because it will make you learn something by the end of everything. So try as much as you can and don't fear losing anything. Don't be afraid of failing because you can't learn anything new with this thinking in life.

Imagine you are on a vacation. You don't have enough time to take in all the sights, sounds and experiences of a foreign land. Wouldn't you thing exactly what you want to do and what you want to miss? And if in mind, you have some fascinating sights and landmarks that you want to visit; wouldn't you do a little research to get to know about their location etc.? Or would you rather just roam around, hoping to find that place eventually on your way?

Similarly, life is exactly like a vacation where you get many opportunities and chances but it depends on you whether to avail them or just let them go easily. But that doesn't mean there is no serendipity in your vacation. During your journey, you'd find many interesting things to experience but it will just make you learn more about yourself and the world you inhabit. But without a clear sense of what you want to do and where you want to go, you would never be able to reach your destination.

Most of us know what our heart yearns for, but we are afraid to go after it. It is often the thing you're afraid of doing but desperately want to do that is your passion and purpose in life. I remember a few years ago I was afraid that I had nothing to contribute to the world with my writing. I was afraid that I wasn't good enough. As the years passed, I became sick of my excuses and negative thoughts, like a kid who stands up to his bully, I decided to stand up to myself and take action anyway.

I wasn't going to let anything stand in my way of doing what I love. If people didn't like it, that was their problem, I was going to do it anyway. And as I started writing; dozens of people read and responded to my writing. And right now, tens of thousands of people read my content every single month. The fears and doubts you have about going after your passion are unfounded. They are there to challenge you to see if you're truly serious about living a happy and fulfilling life. When you are ready to take that step into the unknown even though you are scared, your life will transform. There is a way for you to live a passionate life. I know, because I am living proof.

CHAPTER NINE ENJOY THE JOURNEY

"The journey is the reward."~ Chinese proverb

Once you start accomplishing your goal, you focus on the result you will get at the end but if you pay attention on the achievements you'd discover while getting there, you will be astound. You will never be the same person once you've achieved your significant goal because the experiences you will gain throughout the process will change you completely and that is what the "journey" has rewarded you with.

If you set the goal on losing twenty pounds and you get there, you will have gained more than the result of looking good and having spiked interest from the opposite gender. Now that is what makes you become a changed person.

When you are working towards a goal, in the midway you often say "I am not good enough yet, but I will be when I reach my goal." This is the major problem with your mindset when you try to find happiness in the milestone that is achieved. "Once I achieve my goal, then I'll be happy and successful." This statement is absolutely wrong because you already are a successful person. You know why? Because you are still working on it and has not given it up yet. You are progressing by leaps and bounds and are getting to learn something new. So commit a process, not a goal.

Instead of worrying about the life-changing goals, keep things simple and reduce stress by focusing on the daily process and sticking to your schedule. What is I say I have to lose 10kgs in 20 days? This sentence already stresses me out. But if I start if without taking such burden and having confidence in myself, I know I will be able to achieve it.

RELEASE THE NEED FOR IMMEDIATE RESULTS: We all must adopt a systems-based mentality by sticking to the process instead of jumping to the final step. For example if you are training at a gym and your goal is to lift 40kgs, you definitely would have to undergo a process by lifting lesser amount of kg on daily basis and eventually moving on to the desired amount but if you expect to lift the desired amount on the first day, then the entire work out will be a failure too.

FALL IN LOVE WITH THE JOURNEY: No one in the world can say that goals are useless. I have found that goals are good for planning your progress and systems are good for actually making progress. A well designed journey is the thing that you will always remember for the rest of your life more than the goal which has been achieved. Having a good system is what matters the most and committing to the process is what makes the difference.

It is so easy to read stories and proverbs to enjoy the journey while walking towards our goals, nod our head in agreement but never really take it onboard. But a theoretical appreciation of things is not enough; it needs to be practiced by us if we truly agree to the statements we read in our daily routine.

If you chase experiences and not things, those experiences will change you. The wisdom gained will be internalized and that will be your greatest reward.

Chapter Ten Develop intimate relationships

Having intimate relationship with someone in your life is one of the most important things where you share a sense of closeness and togetherness with another person. This type of relationship between two people usually takes some time to build. It can be made with anyone in the world, parents, friends, cousins, family, or any man or a woman.

When we are young, we make compatible relationship with our parents, we get close to them are learn more and more about them. We love them and feel complete with them but as we grow up, we get a chance to interact with different people of the world. We see variety of people. Some become our favorites while some we hate. We make new friends outside, boyfriend, girlfriend and so many other relations and start establishing commitment and trust with them. We build up connections with other people through work, school, play, sexual contact; parenting etc. the journey towards creating affectionate relationships is therefore potentially never ending.

Sometimes you find a person with all the qualities and feel complete with him while other times there is a certain group of people possessing different qualities in them and you feel comfortable while you are with all of them. So there are different levels of intimacy;

- **Emotional intimacy:** Such a type where you are emotionally attached to a person. You share every type of feelings whether positive or negative with him without having any fear because you are emotionally connected to him.
- **Spiritual intimacy:** When are linked to someone spiritually. We respect them with their beliefs and spiritual needs and understand how spirituality works in their lives.
- **Physical intimacy:** A person who can fulfill you fulfill your physical desires exactly how you want it to be. He gives you a feeling of joy and relaxation by being playful, sensual or sexual.
- **Work intimacy:** You are able to share your work load with that person. And feel completely relieved when he's your partner for the tasks assigned.

- **CRISIS INTIMACY:** You are able to support that person through the time of thick and thin and get over the phase crisis by supporting each other.
- **INTELLECTUAL INTIMACY:** Sharing ideas or discussing issue with each other and still respecting the other person's views and beliefs.

HOW TO BUILD AND MAINTAIN A FAITHFUL RELATIONSHIP?

Everyone wants to build such an intimate relationship that could last forever but only a few works out. Why is that so? People just jump into such relation without knowing how to work on them which results in the separation with their loved ones. Here are some ways that can help you build and maintain a relationship;

PAY ATTENTION TO YOUR PARTNER IN THE EARLY STAGE:

WHEN WE START BUILDING A relationship, we just notice the good things our partner possesses. This is because in the start of every relationship every person tries to be at his/her best. They try to show their positive side only be at their best. They tell the edited version of their life histories but with time they start unmasking themselves which creates a problem for us. That is when the real problem begins.

We had accepted them the way they were in the initial days and later on it becomes a problem for us to be with them due to their changing behavior. But that does simply not mean to leave them and no on. It is our fault who couldn't recognize our partner initially. So we must learn to know a man in the earlier stages before it gets too late. We should try our best to get the most out of him by playing a bit smartly and getting to know every side of him.

OVERT CRITICISM IN A RELATIONSHIP: appreciation is one important factor that every relationship must have. We should avoid every type of negatives thoughts for that person and notice how the qualities of that person. Make him feel good about everything he does and trying not to disagree with him but disapprovals are a part of every relationship too. If your partner is not in a good mood today or is showing you tantrums just think of how well is he overall. A single day should not ruin his overall personality.

SHARE MUTUAL GOALS AND PLANS WITH YOUR PARTNER: In the start of every relationship, try to share and make some mutual goals and plans with your life. What we often do is just about ourselves. How is my life going to be? How much will I enjoy? And everything affiliated to only yourself while the appropriate thing is that once you are with someone then it should become us. You must think about both of you together by keeping his ideas and views in mind too. And this all should be finalized in the initial days of relationships as it becomes a cause of separation late on.

EQUAL GIVE AND TAKE INTERACTION: Try to share equality in your relationship. Give him as much as he is giving you and make him feel special equally. The mindset of women is very typical. They think it's the right of every man to spend on her and buy her everything she wants in the world. Fulfill all her dreams and wishes she has. But men expect something from their ladies too. They want to feel special too. They want their girl to give him equal importance as he is giving to her.

BALANCE IN LIFE: One mistake that almost everyone make is that they lose the balance of commitments in their life over relationships. And once they realize the importance of other things too, the other partner finds it difficult to adjust. So just make sure you maintain a balance in your relationship and other personal conflicts that can promote happiness and longevity to your life.

Chapter Eleven Exercise-An important thing if life

Everyone knows the importance of exercise in our daily routine but there is hardly anyone who knows why is it important. There is a term, "use it, or lose it." It goes exactly for our body. If we don't use our body properly, we will lose it badly. Our muscles will become weak and flabby and all the organs will stop doing their function properly.

Our bodies are deigned to be in motion and active all the time because we have evolved from nomadic ancestors who spent all their time moving from one place to another in search of food and shelter. People develop problems if they sit all day long in front of television or on desk doing nothing and minimize the amount of exercise they do.

Exercise is beneficial mentally as well as physically. Exercise makes you feel fit and active. You feel that you have accomplished something that was hard to strive for. Physical activity gives you more energy and helps you in copying with laziness.

Exercise can be helpful for us in various and abundant ways. Some of its advantages are listed as below,

Prevent diseases: Our bodies are designed to be active and actually crave for exercise. Regular exercise is very important for our physical fitness as it helps to reduce the risk of heart attack, cancer, high blood pressure, diabetes and many other diseases.

Improves stamina: Exercise improves the body stamina by consuming lesser of energy for the same amount of work done. Exercise uses the energy to keep going.

Strengthens and tones: Exercising with weights and other forms of training equipment develops your muscles, bones and ligaments for increased strength and endurance. Posture becomes straight and improved and muscles become more firm. Its helps in making you look better too. So what are you waiting for?

INCREASES FLEXIBILITY: Stretching is another important form of exercise that can help you improve your posture. They keep your body limber which helps you in bending and twisting. It also improves balance and coordination and reduces the chance of injury.

CONTROLS WEIGHT: Working out helps to burn the calories and make you smarter. If you burn off more calories than you take in, you lose weight. It's as simple as that.

IMPROVES QUALITY OF LIFE: Regular exercise can help you improve the living standard of your life. It reduces stress, lifts moods, and helps you sleep better. It makes you free from all the diseases and helps you lead a better life.

IMPROVED SEX LIFE: Exercise makes you feel in shape and tired less that can improve your physical intimacy. It can also enhance the arousal for women and prevents the erectile dysfunction in men.

YOU WILL LIVE LONGER: It's no secret that healthy living will keep you live longer, but you might be surprised at how much. One study found that exercise improves life expectancy as much as quitting smoking. It really is true that sitting all day is killing you—and just a bit of regular exercise can stave off the reaper for a while.

LOWERS TYPE 2 DIABETES RISK. There is an increase in the lower type 2 diabetes across the world but if you don't care about the world, you should care about your own self. By engaging in regular exercise, you improve your body's ability to metabolize glucose, the key to staving off this disease.

MAINTAINS IMMUNE FUNCTIONING. Your immune system is what protects you from infection and other chemical toxins. Short-term exercise programs can reverse some of the deleterious effects of aging on this sensitive and crucial regulatory system which controls so much of your everyday health.

REDUCES THE RISK OF ARTHRITIS THE most commonly experienced chronic illness in middle-aged and older adults, arthritis occurs due to abnormalities in the cartilage and outgrowth of bones in the joints. Unlike the other physical benefits of exercise, reducing the chances of arthritis doesn't depend on heavy duty aerobic activity or even weight training. In fact, you may actually heighten your risk of arthritis if you do too much of the wrong kind of exercise. Running on the pavement, particularly in shoes that aren't appropriately cushioned, can cause you to be more likely to get arthritis. Instead, you need to engage in stretching and flexibility training through yoga, Tai Chi, or other ways to increase the range of movement of your joints. This will lower your risk of injury through muscle tears or torn ligaments, and in the process protect your joints from damage caused by overuse.

BOOSTS MEMORY: Exercise helps your neurons stay in shape particularly in the memory areas of your brain. You don't even have to exert yourself that much to experience this memory boost. Normal walking can help the hippocampus to improve the heath. It also lowers cortisol, the stress hormone, associated with the improved mood and anxiety level.

LOWERS DEMENTIA RISK: Exercise lowers your chances for developing dementia based on cardiovascular illness because you're improving the flow of blood through exercise. Because dementia due to cardiovascular disease is hard to distinguish from other forms of dementia, it's hard to say that exercise could actually slow or prevent the neuron death responsible for Alzheimer's disease. Exercise prevents from Alzheimer's disease by improving your glucose and fat metabolism because some of the brain alterations found in Alzheimer's disease may be due to abnormalities in these processes. It's possible that lack of a healthy lifestyle may have led the illness to develop in many older adult sufferers today. To the extent that middle-agers are now more likely to exercise than were their parents, we may actually see fewer people developing dementia in the coming years.

AEROBIC EXERCISE

Heart enjoys a good workout too exactly like the rest of the muscles. And it can be done the best through aerobic exercise. It is such a type of exercise that improves the pumping of heart and quickens breathing. By giving such a type of work out to heart of regular basis, it can improve the muscles of heart by making them stronger and flexible and affording the pressure the blood makes to it often. If you are playing any sort of sport, you are improving your health and fitness in every way possible. You are making yourself and your body the best for every situation. But if you don't play team sports, don't worry — there are plenty of ways to get aerobic exercise on your own. These include biking, running, swimming, dancing, in-line skating, tennis, cross-country skiing, hiking, and walking quickly. In fact, the types of exercise that you do on your own are easier to continue when you leave high school and go on to work or college, making it easier to stay fit later in life as well. So just make sure you are involved in either type of activity in your life because it gives you betterment in every possible way and is useful for you and your body.

Conclusion

At the outset, this book posed the questions, "What is Endometriosis and how to extinguish it?", "What is happiness and how to live lightheartedly?" and "How to lose weight and live a healthy and an active life?" It is very important to acknowledge this disease as social and communal disease and at the same time recognize its symptoms and affects to fight against endometriosis and live a perfect life without any worries. It also teaches us of staying cognitively sharp with exercise and a healthy diet which is an important way to improve mood and depression, alleviate attention deficits and addiction and relieve stress and anxiety. When explaining stress, exercise makes our bodies and minds stronger and resilient and makes them better for handling future challenges. Regular aerobic activity is also important as it /calms the body.

Printed in Great Britain
by Amazon